TOP

FITNESS

A D V I C E

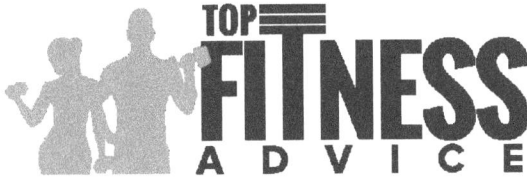

SLEEP YOUR WAY TO GOOD HEALTH

7 Steps to Make TONIGHT The Best Night of Sleep You Have EVER HAD! (And How Sleep Makes You Live Longer & Happier)

Amy Jenkins

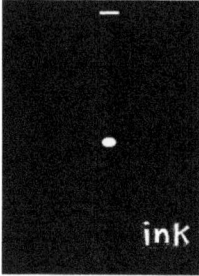

First published in 2017 by Venture Ink Publishing

For more information about the contents of this book or questions to the author, please contact Amy Jenkins at amy@topfitnessadvice.com

Disclaimer

This book provides wellness management information in an informative and educational manner only, with information that is general in nature and that is not specific to you, the reader. The contents of this book are intended to assist you and other readers in your personal wellness efforts. Consult your physician regarding the applicability of any information provided in this book to you.

Nothing in this book should be construed as personal advice or diagnosis, and must not be used in this manner. The information provided about conditions is general in nature. This information does not cover all possible uses, actions, precautions, side-effects, or interactions of medicines, or medical procedures. The information in this book should not be considered as complete and does not cover all diseases, ailments, physical conditions, or their treatment.

You should consult with your physician before beginning any exercise, weight loss, or health care program. This book should not be used in place of a call or visit to a competent health-care professional. You should consult a health care professional before adopting any of the suggestions in this book or before drawing inferences from it.

Any decision regarding treatment and medication for your condition should be made with the advice and consultation of a qualified health care professional. If you have, or suspect you have, a health-care problem, then you should immediately contact a qualified health care professional for treatment.

No Warranties: The author and publisher don't guarantee or warrant the quality, accuracy, completeness, timeliness, appropriateness or suitability of the information in this book, or of any product or services referenced in this book.

The information in this book is provided on an "as is" basis and the author and publisher make no representations or warranties of any kind with respect to this information. This book may contain inaccuracies, typographical errors, or other errors.

Table of Contents

Would you prefer to listen to my book, rather than read it?

Download the audiobook version for free!

If you go to the special link below and sign up to Audible as a new customer, you can get the audiobook version of my book completely free.

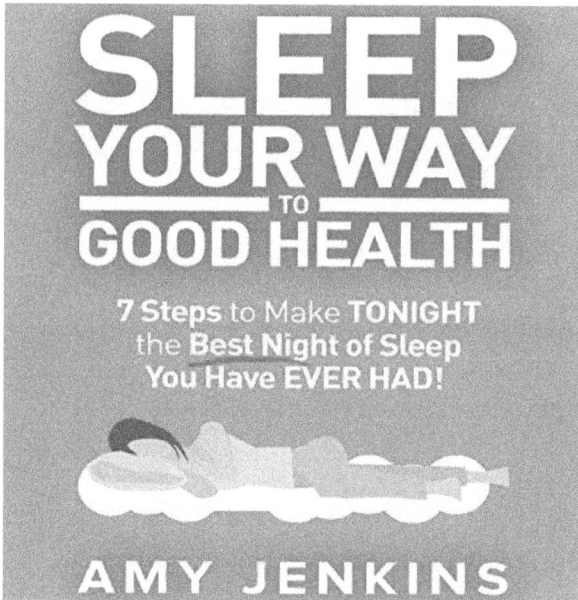

Go here to get your audiobook version for free:

TopFitnessAdvice.com/go/Sleep

Who is this book for?

This book is for those people who battle to get a good night's rest. Whether you battle to fall asleep or you simply cannot seem to sleep enough, you will benefit by reading this book.

Did you know that as much as a third of Americans have trouble when it comes to restful sleep?

And it's not just about getting the right number of hours when it comes to sleep either, truly restorative sleep is something that can be quite elusive.

The good news is that a good sleep pattern is a habit that can be learned like any other.

If you have to rely on the alarm clock to wake up in the morning, or if you need to constantly hit the snooze button, this book is for you.
Look at this book as a master class in getting more restful sleep.

What will this book teach you?

In this book, you will learn what the link between sleep and longevity is and how sleep affects your health, your brain, your weight and your development.

I will explain what sleep hygiene is and explain steps that you can take today to make sure that you are practicing good sleep hygiene.

We go through the importance of complete darkness when it comes to sleep and how you can use sounds and music to help you sleep.

We look at the top natural remedies that will help you start sleeping better tonight and every night that you need them.

We go through how to prepare your mind for the process of falling asleep so that you can get your best possible night's rest.

We look at how to change your diet so that you sleep better at night and how you can break the cycle of sleepless nights that you currently find yourself in.

We look at how to determine how much sleep you really need and how to deal with those nights when sleep just won't come at all.

Introduction

Do you lie awake every night, watching the clock and wishing you could fall asleep? Do you eventually fall asleep only to wake up feeling as though you have not slept in months? Does it feel like, no matter how much sleep you get, you never feel rested?

If so, you are not alone. Millions of Americans are in the same boat. For many of us, poor sleep quality or lack of sleep is a part of everyday life. And is it any surprise? Every day we are expected to do more and more. We have to have it all – it is not uncommon for people to work fourteen-hour days, seven days a week.

And what do we want to do when we get home? Sit in front of the TV and check Facebook all night.

Human beings were designed to get up when the sun came up and go to bed when the sun went down. Most of us, however, don't want to miss out. And with all the advancements in technology we don't have to. We can watch every funny cat video on the internet and stay up until dawn if we want to.

We can have it all – and a helping of insomnia on the side. Never in our history have sleep aids been so widely available. And never in our history have we been so sleep deprived.

Are you ready to break the cycle? Are you ready to get some sleep? To feel rested and well for the first time in ages?

If you are ready to turn your back on sleeplessness, this book is for you. Start sleeping better from tonight with these simple and inexpensive tips. Start the journey to a whole new you today.

Discover Scientifically-Proven "Shortcuts" & "Hacks" to Lose Weight FASTER (With Very Little Effort)

For this month only, you can get Linda Westwood's best-selling & most popular book absolutely free – *Weight Loss Secrets You NEED to Know.*

Get Your FREE Copy Here:

TopFitnessAdvice.com/Extras

Discover scientifically-proven tips to help you lose weight faster and easier than ever before. With this book, readers were able to improve their weight loss results and fitness levels. So, it's highly recommended that you get this book, especially while it's free!

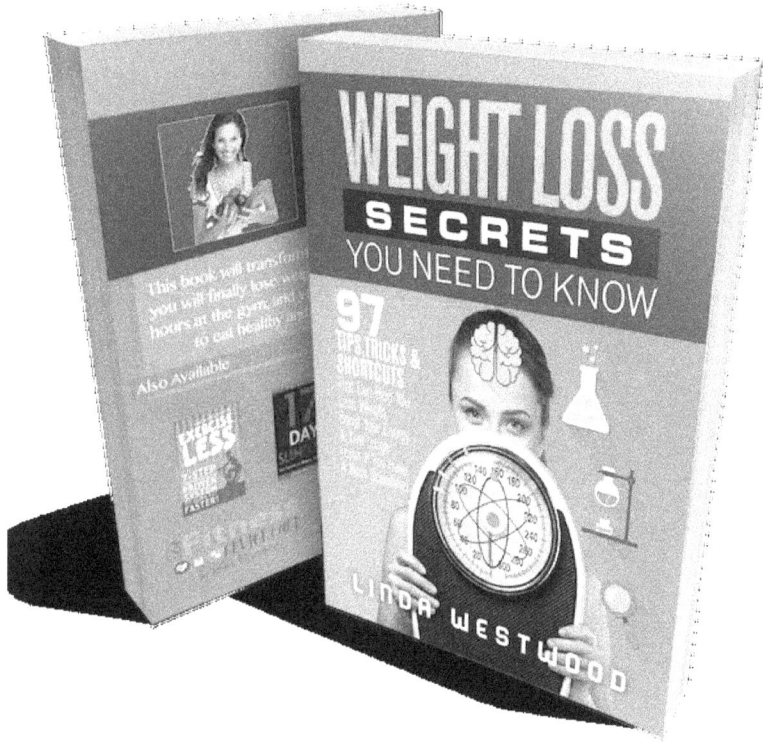

Get Your FREE Copy Here:

TopFitnessAdvice.com/Extras

Sleep and Longevity

Research has shown that sleeping too little, or too much, has a significant impact on your expected lifespan.

According to a study that tracked 21,000 twins over a period of 22 years, seven to eight hours a night is ideal. This can differ from one individual to the next.

The study focused on twins because they would have the same backgrounds and genetic makeup.

The study looked at how well they slept, how long they slept and whether or not they used medication to sleep.

It was found that those participants who slept for longer than eight hours or less than seven hours a night were 17%-24% more likely to die earlier. It was also found that those using medications to sleep had an increased mortality risk of around a third.

Why Is Sleep So Important?

During sleep, the body carries out necessary repairs. Being sleep-deprived short-circuits this process and places the body under unnecessary stress.

This affects all the systems in the body. Sleep deprivation can cause hypertension and cardiac disease, contribute to the development of diabetes, cause depression, and an increase in body weight.

In the next chapter, we will go through all of these in more detail but for now, it suffices to say that lack of quality sleep over an extended period can have serious side effects when it comes to your health.

The diseases that can develop as a result of sleep deprivation can have a significant impact on both your quality of life and your longevity as a whole.

Sleep and Your Health

Longevity is not the only casualty when you are not getting enough sleep.

Sleep and Mental Health

The way that you think and feel is significantly impacted by how well you sleep.

During sleep, the brain helps to order and process information that you have learned during the day. Your subconscious makes sense of what has happened to you and your conscious mind gets to take a break.

Without enough sleep, your brain is not able to process this information as it should. This affects your memory and your ability to deal with your emotions. Sleep deficiency over time impacts your problem-solving abilities and your creativity as well.

When you are deprived of sleep, your mind is automatically less able to deal with stress. You are also more likely to feel depressed and unable to cope.

Sleep and Your Brain

Studies have also shown a worrying link between sleep deprivation and the death of brain cells. It was found that even one episode of bad sleep could result in the loss of brain tissue.

MRIs revealed that those who chronically lost sleep suffered more rapid decline of brain function than those who were well-rested.

Sleep and Your Physical Health

If you do not get enough sleep, your body is unable to complete the repairs that it needs to. Sleep deprivation puts the immune system under pressure and makes it less able to deal with infections.

Not getting enough sleep makes you more likely to suffer a stroke, develop cardiac disease, hypertension and diabetes.

Sleep and Your Weight

If you battle to stick to a diet because you want to eat everything in sight, it could be that you are sleep-deprived. When your body does not get the energy reserves it needs from a good night's sleep, it needs to get them from food.

If you have a bad night's sleep, production of the hormones that control hunger become unbalanced.

Levels of ghrelin increase so that you feel hungrier and eat more. Levels of leptin are decreased so that you do not feel as full as you should after eating.

You are also less able to make good food choices and the combination of these three factors is deadly for your weight.

Sleep and Growth and Development

In children, a lack of deep sleep interferes with the production of growth hormone. This interferes with the development of proper muscle and bone growth in children.

Sleep and Your Safety and Performance

Those who are sleep deprived are slower to respond to external stimuli. This can negatively impact your safety as you are not able to act quickly enough to avoid an accident.

In addition, those who have lost sleep are less productive overall and more prone to making mistakes.

After a few nights losing sleep, even as little as an hour or so a night, your daily functioning ability is affected as much as if you had not slept at all the previous night.

And if it carries on, your brain might go into micro-sleep mode. This is where you fall asleep, even just for a minute or two, whatever you are doing. You might not even remember falling asleep.

I hope that you are enjoying this book so far, and if you could spare 30 seconds, I would greatly appreciate you leaving a review on Amazon.com.

The Importance of Good Sleep Hygiene

Sleep can be very elusive. It seems as though the more we chase after it, the harder it can be to catch.

With the advent of electric lights and advances in technology, we no longer need to follow the natural cycles of nature. We were designed to wake with the sun and go to sleep when the sun goes down.

As the light dims in the evening, our bodies begin to produce melatonin and this, in turn, helps get us ready for sleep.

When we are exposed to the bright daylight, melatonin production is stopped and we wake up fully.

The problem now is that the electric lights we use and the light emitted by the screens of our appliances such TVs and phones have a similar effect to daylight.

Our sleep patterns become more and more disrupted because we are effectively exposed to what our bodies perceive as daylight for longer.

What is Sleep Hygiene?

The term "sleep hygiene" can seem a little confusing. You might wonder what hygiene has to do with sleep at all.

In this context, it means establishing a routine and environment that are conducive to sleep.

Sleep hygiene covers the following:

- Making your bedroom dark enough to sleep
- Cutting out extraneous noises
- Ensuring that your bedroom is a comfortable temperature
- Making sure that your bed offers firm support
- Establishing a set bed-time routine, including a "wind-down" stage
- Waking up at the same time every day
- Associating your bed with sleep and sex only

Good Sleep Hygiene

It's important because it makes it a lot easier for you to fall asleep. Your body gets into an established routine and this supports the proper release of melatonin.

Your body has an environment that supports the sleep process making it easier to fall asleep and to get a good night's sleep.

Turn Out the Lights

Light has an extremely disruptive effect on sleep because it can block the production of melatonin in the body.

As mentioned before, electric lights have the same effect as daylight when it comes to melatonin production. If you want to get a great night's sleep, you need to ensure that your bedroom is as dark as possible.

Banish the TV

It is time to say goodbye to the TV in your bedroom. For those that believe that they must have the TV in the background in order to fall asleep, this is a tough one.

Maybe you've convinced yourself that you must watch TV until you fall asleep. The truth is though that this is more of a habit and could be hampering your attempts at a good night's rest.

Who of us is not guilty of the odd Netflix binge? How often have you said to yourself that you will just watch one more episode?

How often has "just one more episode" turned into five or more? The TV is very stimulating for the mind. The light it emits and the programs that you are watching keep the mind active long after you switch off. You need to switch the TV off at least an hour before you go to bed.

Get Rid of The Phone

Your phone is just as bad as the TV when it comes to keeping your mind active. Even if you have it set to bedside mode so it doesn't ping, the phone can still be a big distraction.

Checking your phone "one last time" can end up waking you up and damage your chances of falling asleep. You need to be brutal here. Switch your phone off at least an hour before bedtime and don't look at it again until you wake up in the morning.

Check for LED Lights

When I moved into a new house, I had trouble sleeping for the longest time. I couldn't understand it, I had done everything I could to make the room dark, control external noise, temperature, etc.

In theory, I should have been able to sleep. It wasn't until I had some really bad nights that I began to realize that the room was not really completely dark, despite my efforts. I looked for the source of the light

Our house's alarm system was plugged into the electrical outlet under the vanity in my room. It had a green LED light that was always on. Now, this glow was partially obscured by the vanity but it still gave off a lot of light at night.

I found a way to cover that light at night and started to sleep a lot better. If you do have any electrical appliances in your room, check for standby lights that are on all the time. The light from these can be surprisingly bright on a dark night.

If you have an electric alarm clock with the time lit up by LED lighting, this is just as bad. In fact, it might even be worse because the light keeps you awake and you are easily able to see how late it is getting. Clear out any source of light in your bedroom as a whole.

Black-out Blinds

These are an inexpensive way to ensure that you get a better night's sleep. I always have a layer of black-out material sewn into the lining of my curtains.

I also have a set of blinds that hang in the window in addition to the curtains. This makes such a difference when it comes to getting a good night's sleep because it blocks out any light coming from outside.

A Sleeping Mask

A sleeping mask can provide an extra layer of protection against the dark to ensure that you get a great night's sleep.

Try to find one made from natural fibers like cotton so that air can still circulate near the skin.

I made my own out of cotton toweling because those made from polyester make my skin feel hot and sweaty.

Once again, thank you for reading this book, and I hope you're getting a lot of valuable information. I would greatly appreciate it if you could take 30 seconds to leave me a review for this book on Amazon.com.

Sound to Help You Sleep

Ideally, the quieter your environment is when you sleep the better it is for you. Loud sounds are detrimental to sleep because they can stimulate the brain.

On the other hand, relaxing, repetitive sounds can help you to fall asleep faster as they are soothing. Sound can help you sleep by drowning out other disruptive sounds and by helping your mind to relax.

You should look for sounds or music that have no lyrics. If you can sing along to the tune, it might prove disruptive to sleep. You want it to play softly in the background – loud enough so that you can hear it but not so loud that it actually keeps you awake.

What Do You Find Soothing?

This is largely a matter of personal preference. Let us look at classical music, for example. If you love listening to it, it might be very soothing for you and could help you sleep.

If you hate classical music, however, you are more likely to find it disruptive.

What I advise is that you try a range of different sounds to see what you personally find relaxing. In this chapter, we'll go through some of your options.

White Noise

White noise machines are quite a popular option. The sound is not music at all but more of a masking tone. It helps to drown out annoying noises.

It is best to use a white noise machine or download something from a site such as **www.simplynoise.com**.

Nature Sounds

Sounds of nature such as the sound of the ocean, of the rainforest, storms, etc. can be soothing and relaxing. Because they are natural sounds, they are less likely to be annoying.

The repetitive sound of waves breaking on the beach can be extremely soothing. Do try it out first though because sounds that include water might cause you to want to go to the bathroom.

Music

If you are worried about something, music can help you to relax. Do be careful about listening to music that has lyrics as this may be more stimulating. Stick to music that has a slower tempo and be sure to set the timer so that it switches off after about twenty minutes or so.

Whilst the sound might help you to fall asleep, it could end up disrupting the deeper sleep patterns later in the night so it's better not to play it all night.

Relaxation CDS

Some of these are pretty good. They are similar to guided meditations in that they read out a set of instructions to help you relax. Choose a voice that you find soothing for best results.

Natural Remedies to Help You Sleep

It can be very distressing not to be able to sleep, especially if it has been happening for several nights in a row. Some people turn to their doctors for help and are prescribed sleeping tablets.

I will caution you not to turn to prescription medication unless there is absolutely no option. If you do decide to take it, it should be viewed as a very short-term measure. And by that, I mean less than a week.

Sleeping tablets have been proven to be highly addictive and prevent you from reaching the deeper, more restorative stages of sleep. It is far better to try natural remedies or adjusting your diet before you try sleeping tablets.

In this chapter, we will go through some of the myriad of home remedies out there. Don't be too discouraged if some of these do not work for you – something will, you may just need to experiment to find out what that is for you.

Just one note here, when it comes to things that you take internally, like valerian, catnip tea, etc. it can be tempting to take double quantities just to "make sure" it works. Resist the urge to do so – natural remedies taken to excess can be just as dangerous as prescription medication. Start with the lowest possible dose and increase that only of necessary.

Unsweetened Cherry Juice

As little as a half cup of unsweetened cherry juice can help you to fall asleep. It contains a lot of the amino acid Tryptophan, the precursor to serotonin and melatonin. Drink half a cup or a full cup about an hour before you want to go to sleep.

Clear the Clutter

Making sure that your bedroom is clean and tidy can go a long way to promoting sleep. Even if you no longer really notice the clutter consciously, research has shown that it still affects you sub-consciously.

Valerian

Valerian is an herbal remedy that has been used for centuries as a natural sleep aid. It has a calming effect on the body and mind and increases the amount of GABA available to the brain. This enables you to relax and sleep better.

It has a similar action to sleeping tablets in that it increases the amount of GABA available to the brain but it differs in that it does not interfere with the restorative phase of sleep.

It is possible to get hooked on valerian, though not to the same extent as sleeping tablets. It is therefore advisable to give it a break if using it daily for more than two weeks. You can take it in the form of tablets, a tincture or a tea. Choose whatever is easiest for you.

Acupuncture

Okay, so this is not strictly a home treatment but it is a natural option that can be helpful. Acupuncture can help clear energy blockages within the body and this can help your overall nervous system and physical health as well.

Lower Your Body Temperature

Part of the process that the body undergoes when preparing for sleep is to reduce the body temperature. You can use this to your advantage if you want to induce sleep.

A nice warm bath about an hour before bedtime will relax the muscles and also raise your body temperature. The temperature will drop off after that leaving you feeling sleepy.

There are also those who advocate putting on a pair of cool, damp socks to achieve the same effect but I must say that the warm bath appeals to me better.

In summer, when you are feeling the heat, a cool bath or shower can be just as helpful when it comes to lowering your core temperature.

Herbal Tea

Chamomile, Passion Flower and Hops teas are all great aids to help you sleep. You can make up a blend of all three if you like. Take a tablespoon each of the dried herb and pour boiling water over it.

Let it steep for at least 10-15 minutes. Drink the tea about a half an hour to an hour before going to bed.

Catnip and Skullcap can also be useful herbs to help you sleep but they do not taste all that good. You can sweeten the tea with a little honey if you prefer.

Having a cup of tea as part of your nightly routine will help you settle into a routine that lets your body know it is time to sleep. Drink your tea at the same time every night to help cement your routine.

Melatonin Supplementation

Taking a melatonin supplement has been found useful for some people in promoting a better quality of sleep. Research found that it was not effective for everyone though.

The jury is out on this one but it may be better to eat foods rich in tryptophan rather than supplementing with melatonin. Tryptophan is needed by the body to produce serotonin and that is needed to produce melatonin. Cherries, bananas, chicken/ turkey and milk are all rich in tryptophan.

Bananas

It may seem a little strange but bananas are the ideal sleep-time snack. They are rich in tryptophan and magnesium, both necessary for calming the body. They also have some protein and fiber in them to help you feel fuller.

Finally, they are rich in carbs which are also helpful in making you feel more relaxed. Have a banana half an hour before you want to go to sleep.

Exercise

There are some relaxing stretches that you can do before going to bed to help your body relax. Regular exercise also helps you to reduce your stress levels and helps your body to function as it should. It improves your overall health and vitality and can help to reduce niggling aches and pains.

That said, cardio exercise can rev up your energy levels so you should not do any cardio within four hours of going to bed. Stick with gentle stretching or a simple relaxation exercise before bed.

A Peace Pillow

Peace pillows are not as popular as they once were and this is a pity because they can be very effective. All you need to do is to make a small pillow that can fit inside your normal pillow case. Use natural fibers for this or use a very thin sock.

Fill it with the leaves and flowers of dried lavender and place inside your pillow case. Do not use the stalks as these can be quite hard and can poke you.

Place the peace pillow just inside the top cover of the pillow case so that you will be able to smell the lavender. The lavender is crushed when you lie on it, releasing its scent.

If you cannot get hold of dried lavender, you can use lavender essential oil instead by just dropping two or three drops on your pillow case. Personally, I prefer the peace pillow because I find that the scent is not quite as strong as that of the essential oil.

Aromatherapy Oils

Aromatherapy can be very effective at helping you to sleep. As mentioned above, I find the scent of Lavender essential oil a little too strong for my liking but try it, you may not. It is a very relaxing oil to use.

I use a blend of oils instead – I use equal parts of sandalwood and neroli oil. To that I add half the amount of ylang-ylang oil. (Ylang-ylang can be over-powering so go slowly when using it.)

There are many ways to use the essential oils. You can drop them into your bath or diffuse them in your room. You can drop them onto a tissue and place that inside your pillow case if you like.

Alternatively, you can mix them into an aqueous cream or sweet almond oil and apply them directly to the body. Keep the dilutions to a maximum of 2% - the oils are very concentrated and can burn your skin if applied neat.

Eat Some Carbs

Considering the popularity of low carb diets and banting, this may sound like sacrilege but carbs are necessary to help the body and brain process tryptophan more easily. The ideal before bed snack is a high-carb food item like bread or a banana and with a little protein, like some turkey or a little milk.

Magnesium

This is one mineral that the body needs the most and yet it is the one that we are most likely to be deficient in. The typical Western diet is low in magnesium and high in refined foods.

Leafy greens are amongst the richest sources of magnesium in the diet and something that few of us get enough of. Magnesium is especially important when it comes to the GABA receptors in your brain. GABA is essential when it comes to calming your nervous system.

If you feel that you may be deficient in magnesium, taking a supplement at night with supper or about an hour before bed can help.

Magnesium is a mineral that is better absorbed through the skin so you could also try a topical application of magnesium. (Try your local health store to find a spray or oil that you can use.)

A very simple and inexpensive way to get more magnesium and to help the muscles relax at the same time is to have a hot bath with Epsom salts added to it. Please note that this is not a good idea if you suffer from high blood pressure or epilepsy.

It is best to do this just before bed time. Add a cup to two cups of Epsom salts to the water, as warm as you can manage, and soak for at least 20 minutes. Keep a glass of water on hand and sip it throughout. Alternatively, make yourself a cup of herbal tea like chamomile tea and drink that.

This helps to relax the muscles, give the body a dose of magnesium and draw toxins out. You can add a half cup of baking soda to intensify the detox properties of the bath.

You can also add essential oils such as sandalwood, lavender, chamomile, neroli or ylang-ylang to bolster the soothing effect of the bath.

When you get out of the bath, dry yourself off, wrap yourself up warmly and climb into bed. The bath will cause sweating as well. A nice side effect of the bath is that it softens your skin beautifully.

Lemon Balm

Lemon balm has been used throughout the ages as a cure for an overwrought mind and nervous tension. Lemon Balm, or Melissa, as it is sometimes known is highly beneficial to take as a tea. It helps relax the mind and can ease depression as well.

The herb is easy enough to grow so do put some in the garden if you have space. Where possible, use the fresh herb to make the tea.

Take a quarter cup of the leaves, flowers and stalks and bruise them slightly. Pour boiling water over the top and leave it to steep for 10-15 minutes. You can add honey if you want to sweeten it a bit.

Alternatively, you can use about half the quantity of the dried herb. If you cannot get hold of the herb, the essential oil can be quite useful as well.

Do NOT drink the essential oil but use it in the bath, in a diffuser, on a tissue or in a cream or oil.

St. John's Wort

St. John's Wort is another herbal remedy that can be helpful when dealing with anxiety and depression.

Studies have shown that it can be as effective as prescription anti-depressants in cases of mild to moderate depression. You can drink it as a tea or use a supplement.

Personally, I find that the supplement is a better choice. It will take a little while for you to start seeing results so do be patient.

If you are currently taking prescription anti-depressants, consult your doctor before taking St John's Wort – they should not be taken together.

Hops

No, this is not an excuse to go and have another beer. In this case, you want to use the dried form of the herb. You can either make yourself a cup of hops tea about an hour before bedtime or you can add hops to your peace pillow. The herb promotes a deep and restful sleep.

Warm Milk

A glass of warm milk with a teaspoon of honey in it is an old recipe for helping you sleep. The milk contains tryptophan, calcium and magnesium and this could assist you in falling asleep.

It is probably more effective from a psychological basis in that it is very soothing. Most people remember being given warm milk to help them sleep as a child and so it is a pleasant memory.

Catnip

Wrestle away the catnip from your cats – it is also a good way to treat insomnia when taken in the form of a tea. You will need about a half a cup of the fresh herb or about 2 tablespoons of the dried herb per cup of boiling water.

Now, I do have to caution you – this really does not taste good. Let it steep for 10-15 minutes and then sip it down as fast as you can. You can try to add some honey but it doesn't help much.

Why I have included it here is that it is also helpful for treating colds and flu and a runny stomach. (If you have a runny stomach, double the amount of catnip in your tea.)

I have found that one cup of catnip tea is as effective as over the counter medication when it comes to a runny tummy. If you have a runny tummy and want a good night's sleep, this is the tea for you.

A GABA Supplement

Evidence as to whether supplementation with GABA can help you sleep is mainly anecdotal. There is some concern in the scientific community about whether or not the GABA in this form actually even reaches the brain at all.

Here I can only speak from personal experience. I do find that the GABA supplement helps me to sleep. It helps me to relax, makes me sleepy and I sleep much better when I take it. I also find that I am calmer the next day.

Now, according to science, this could very well be the placebo effect at play. All I can say is that, placebo effect or not, it works for me. What I do suggest is that if you find not much else is working for you, try taking 500mg GABA about half an hour before going to bed.

Empty Your Bladder Before Bedtime

Making sure that your bladder is empty at bedtime may not actually help you fall asleep but it can help you sleep through the night more comfortably.

Make Sure Your Feet are Warm

If you are battling to fall asleep, try checking to make sure that your feet are warm. If the extremities of your body are cold, it can make falling asleep that much more difficult.

I dislike sleeping with socks on but I keep a pair next to my bed. During my wind-down session, I check to see if my feet are cold.

If they are, I put the socks on and take them off again just before I go to sleep.

If you feel comfortable sleeping with socks on, feel free to wear them all night.

Others who are considering purchasing this book would love to know what you think. If you could spare a few seconds, they would greatly appreciate reading an honest review from you. Simply visit the page on Amazon.com.

Preparing Your Mind for Sleep

If you are only going to try one method out of this whole book, then I hope that it is this one. Getting your mind ready for rest is one of the most effective things you can do when it comes to establishing a regular sleep pattern again.

Your body is a creature of habit, it craves routine. By having a set schedule that you follow every night before going to bed, you make things easier for your body. The wind-down ritual becomes a habit – when you have your herbal tea, the body knows bed-time is coming and prepares itself accordingly.

In this chapter, we will go through what you can do to instill this routine.

Dim the Lights

We have already discussed the effect that electric lights have on melatonin production. The best possible thing to do would be to switch all the lights off at sunset and go to bed but that is not very practical, is it?

What you can do is to limit your exposure to the light. Where possible, install lower-wattage bulbs and dimmer switches. The later it gets, the dimmer your lights should get.

Start dimming the lights from about 8 o'clock at least to help your body naturally start getting ready for sleep. Also, make sure that the bathroom light is dimmer so that it won't wake you if you need to use the bathroom during the night.

If you can't install a dimmer switch, there is another method that you can try. Now, I must admit that when I first read about this, I thought it was whacky. I never thought that it would work well at all, but it does.

Ever wondered why some people wear their sunglasses at night? It could be that they have trouble sleeping.

A good pair of sunglasses will have the same effect at night that they do during the day – they cut the glare and intensity of the light. It sounds nuts but it actually works – try it tonight and you'll see for yourself.

Have a Cut-off Time

This one was tough for me – I spend a lot of time on my computer and phone and I know only too well the joys of binge-watching Netflix.

That said, the use of electronic devices is stimulating for your mind. Watching that last TV show does more harm than it does good. The light from the TV, at the very least, prevents your brain from producing enough melatonin.

Switch off all electronic devices at least an hour or two before you want to sleep. If you are using your phone as an alarm, set the alarm and switch off the phone. Set it somewhere that you can't see it straight away.

Switch off the computer, TV, etc. and find something else to do for the hour or so before bed. This could be having a relaxing bath; it could be sitting in a dimly lit room reading – you choose.

You can do whatever you like as long as it does not involve electronics (you can play relaxing music if you want) or anything that is physically or mentally stimulating.

Set Up a Routine

What do you need to do each night before you go to bed? Have a bath/ shower, change into your PJs, brush your teeth, etc.

Start doing these in the same order every night. This reinforces the association that each of these actions have with bedtime. Your body learns the routine – shower, PJ's, Brush Teeth, Read, Sleep and your brain will automatically move into sleep mode at the appropriate time.

Go to Bed When You Are Tired

As babies, we knew this instinctively. As we get older, we keep on worrying more and more that we are going to miss out on something.

Yes, if you force yourself to stay awake, you will probably get a "second wind" and be able to go on for longer. The problem is that this is as a result of your body reacting to what it perceives as a stressful, life or death situation.

In order to keep you awake, your body releases cortisol. This enables you to stay awake for a few hours longer but can come at a great cost.

Your body has to deal with all that excess cortisol so you have a higher resting level of cortisol. This interferes with the levels of other hormones in the blood and makes you feel edgier and more irritable than normal.

It interferes with the way your body responds to insulin and so your body is less able to process the glucose in what you eat. The higher levels of blood sugar mean that the body produces even more insulin and your hormones are even more out of balance.

You feel hungrier and eat more and the cycle keeps repeating itself. If this happens on a regular basis, you run the risk of developing insulin resistance or Type 2 Diabetes.

Cut Out the Late-night Pig-out

What you eat, as you will see in the next chapter, can have an effect on how well you sleep.

Eating a large meal may make you sleepy but it can actually keep you awake as the digestive tract works on processing all that food. Spicy foods can rev up the metabolism and cause indigestion, making it harder to go to sleep.

Drinking too many liquids can make it necessary to get up during the night to use the bathroom. Limit evening food and drinks.

Read a Relaxing Book

Find an author that is easy to read and whose books are relaxing to read rather than exciting.

This is not the time to start reading those page-turners when you have to carry on reading to find out what happened.

Alternatively, find a non-fiction book that you can read. The goal here is to find something that will help you forget about your worries without getting you overly stimulated.

Breathing Exercises

This is a great exercise to help you relax and help your mind switch off for a bit:

- Breathe in deeply for the count of five.
- Hold your breath for the count of five.
- Breathe out for the count of five.
- Repeat until you feel calmer and more relaxed.

During the exercise, all you need to concentrate on is your breathing. This is a kind of meditation that allows you to completely clear your mind.

Gratitude Exercise

Take a little time out just before you drift off to think of the two or three things you are most grateful for in your life. All too often, we are so worried about what we want that we don't focus on what we have.

This exercise will help you feel more relaxed and content within yourself and about what you already do have.

Enjoying this book?

Check out our other best sellers!

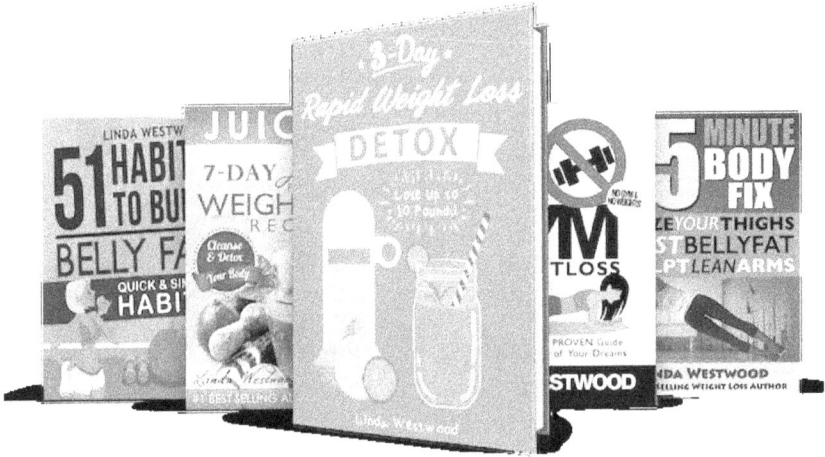

Dietary Changes to Improve Sleep

When it comes to dietary changes, the best thing that you can do is to give your body the nutrition it craves. So many of the little aches and pains that we experience can be attributed to micro-nutrient deficiencies.

Eating a wholefood, balanced diet will help your body to maintain optimal health and this will help you sleep better at night. The timing of meals is important as well.

Eating a good breakfast and lunch makes it less likely that you will overeat at dinner-time. This, in turn, makes it less likely that your sleep will be disturbed by indigestion. Having a balanced diet will also help your body to maintain a balanced blood sugar level and this can also help to improve your chances of sleep.

Have you ever had dinner too early, or skipped it completely only to find that you are unable to sleep? Whilst eating too much before bedtime is bad for your sleep, not eating enough can be just as bad. Your body will make you lie awake until you have a small snack.

Keep a Food Diary

By keeping a thorough food diary, you will be able to see whether or not you have developed any sensitivities to the food you eat

Do you have some kind of gluten- or lactose-intolerance? Take a look at what you ate on those days when you battled to sleep. It could be an undiagnosed food-intolerance that is keeping you awake.

Ditch the Caffeine

And here, I am not just talking about coffee but anything that contains caffeine in general. Tea, chocolates, energy drinks, etc. all contain caffeine and can affect your system for around about 6 hours.

For those who are more sensitive to the effects of caffeine, this period is even longer. To be on the safe side, cut out all caffeine after two in the afternoon. Try alternatives such as herbal teas. Red Bush (or Rooi Bos) tea is a nice-tasting alternative.

Ditch the Refined Sugar

Research has been finding that refined sugar is a lot more dangerous than we ever could have imagined.

We know about its impact on blood sugar and consequent influence on weight but what you might not know is that it can be just as negative when it comes to sleep for the exact same reason.

Eat sugar too close to bedtime and you'll have a sugar-rush that will keep you awake. The consequent sugar crash can have the same effect by making your body crave fuel.

Complex Carbs

Complex carbs are a much better choice when it comes to a snack before bedtime, especially when combined with a little protein.

Other studies have indicated that when you eat the carbs is as important as what carbs you eat. If you are on a low-carb diet, eat most of your carbs with dinner in order to help you sleep faster and better.

Getting Enough B Vitamins

Vitamin B6 is essential when it comes to the body being able to convert tryptophan into serotonin. If you do not get enough B6, your body's ability to produce serotonin may be impacted and your sleep can suffer. Bananas, chickpeas, fish and poultry are rich in B6.

B3 will help you to sleep for longer and sleep more deeply. If you keep waking up throughout the night, it might be as a result of not getting enough B3. Poultry, beets, peanuts and pork are rich in B3.

Watch How Much Alcohol You Drink

Alcohol can help to make you sleepy and so people often resort to drinking if they are unable to sleep. This is counterproductive though – alcohol may make you sleepy but it will disrupt your restorative REM sleep later on in the night.

The effect is that whilst you may fall asleep faster after having a drink or two, you will not sleep as well and will wake up feeling unrefreshed.

I hope you have learned something from this book so far and would greatly appreciate it if you could leave an honest review on Amazon.com.

Resetting Your Sleep Cycle

Resetting your sleep cycle once it is out of whack can be tough but it can be done if you are consistent in your efforts. Now, how long it takes will depend on how bad your sleep cycle has gotten.

Let's say, for example, that you don't feel tired until midnight anymore but you should be going to bed at ten. It is going to take some time to get your body tired in time for bed at ten.

It's also going to possibly mean losing even more sleep, at least in the beginning.

Start Off with Getting Up at the Same Time Every Day

If you want to start resetting your sleep cycle, it is best to start over a weekend or during a time that you are not going to need to be at your very best.

Now it is time to start being very strict with yourself. No matter what time you go to bed, set your alarm for the same time every day.

Ideally, you should aim for eight hours a night so if you get up at six in the morning, you should be asleep by ten at night.

Go through the steps that I have laid out in the book:

- Make sure your room is dark and quiet

- Make sure your bed is comfortable and firm

- Get the temperature of your bedroom right

- Dim the lights early or wear sunglasses in the evening

- Switch off the electronics an hour before bed at the latest

- Have a nice warm bath with a cup of herbal tea of your choice about an hour before bedtime – use essential oils if you like. In summer, a cool shower/ bath is just as effective

- Set up your own nighttime routine

- Settle down to read or do some other task that will relax you and get you ready for sleep

- Go to bed

The next morning, get up as soon as the alarm goes off. There is no snoozing.

Initially, this may be difficult because the chances are good that you wouldn't have fallen asleep at ten the night before. It will take a little while for your body to adjust to the new cycle.

Given time, and consistent effort, it will though. The most important thing is not to change the time that you wake up for any reason. This might mean having to drag yourself through a long few days but your sleep patterns will adjust pretty quickly

Light Up Your Mornings

The next most important thing to do is to expose yourself to natural light as soon as you wake up. Get up and open the curtains. Go for a quick walk outside. This will get your body into wake-up mode a lot more quickly and help to reset your sleep cycle.

Remember how we said that routine was key when it came to a settled sleep cycle? Always make exposure to light part of your early morning routine. It will be more useful at waking you up than having a cup of coffee.

Cut the Stimulants After Twelve

It's not like you will never be able to have a cup of coffee ever again but while you are resetting your sleep cycle, you want to cut out all stimulants that might affect your sleep. This means nothing with caffeine in it after noon. Keep the sugary foods after that to a minimum as well.

Also, have a look at the medication that you are taking – some of it can cause insomnia as a side effect. Can you take that medication in the morning?

If you need the medication for a chronic condition, be sure to speak to a health care professional before changing your dosages. If you are concerned that the medication is causing your insomnia, see if you can get them to change to a different medication.

No Alcohol

Again, I am not saying that you can never drink alcohol again, but during the adjustment period, it is better to steer clear of it completely.

Be Very Strict about Switching Off the TV, Phone, etc.

That awesome tweet that you just thought of will have to wait until tomorrow. Write it down if you really must but do not break the rule about electronics during the adjustment phase.

Once your body gets used to the new routine, this will be easier – you will start to look forward to your unwinding session.

Focus on What You are Gaining

Okay, so maybe you really want to see what happens to your favorite character at the end of your favorite TV show. Maybe you want to surf the internet some more.

Instead of focusing on what you are missing out, look at what it is that you are gaining. Sure, you might not be able to do as much at night anymore but you'll have a lot more time in the morning now.

You'll sleep better and be more able to be productive and healthy. Make sure that you enjoy some aspect of your new routine so that you look forward to it every night again.

Cut Distractions

Does your spouse's snoring keep you awake at night? Perhaps you need to invest in ear plugs or sleep in another room. What other distractions may keep you from falling asleep? Find ways to cut off as many distractions as you can.

No Daytime Naps

Power naps can be useful but while you are resetting your sleep cycle, you are more likely to find that naps are disruptive. Don't give in to the temptation to nap during the day. It may feel good initially but will just set you back.

Cut Yourself Some Slack

Okay, so you did everything right, you turned off all the electronics, did the whole routine and everything and you still aren't able to fall asleep. Cut yourself some slack.

There are going to be times when that happens. Don't make a big deal out it. Don't check the time and worry that you are going to be like a zombie in the morning.

Fun fact: If you fall asleep as soon as your head hits the pillow, you are probably sleep deprived. It is normal to take about 15 minutes or so to fall asleep.

Get Started

One of the hardest things about resetting your sleep schedule is to get started. You know that you are probably in for a few bad night's sleep. You don't want to be tired and cranky. Maybe you'll start next week instead.

The sooner you get it started, the sooner you will be able to finish it. Examine why you want to put off resetting your sleep schedule.

If you have an important presentation coming up in the next couple of days, by all means put off starting. If you just don't want to be tired and cranky, stop making excuses and get it over and done with.

Don't Let Mistakes Trip You Up

You are bound to make a mistake or two along the way. Maybe you hit the snooze button or maybe you sleep through the alarm.

Again, cut yourself a break and move on. One or two slipups along the way are not going to invalidate all your efforts. Using those slipups as a reason to give up and fall back into old routines, however, will cancel out all the hard work that you have done.

How Much Sleep Do You Need?

Your ultimate aim should be to ditch the alarm clock altogether. If you need an alarm clock to wake you every morning, you are not getting enough sleep. Once your sleep pattern has become more entrenched, you can start tweaking it by adding more sleeping time if you need it. Start by putting your bed-time routine ahead by 15 minutes so that you end up going to bed 15 minutes earlier.

Once you have settled into that cycle, check if you still need the alarm clock to wake you in the mornings. If you do, repeat the process. This way you can be sure that you are getting the rest that your body needs.

On the other hand, if you find that you are consistently waking up a bit before the alarm goes off, you probably don't need as much sleep. Get up and start your day when you wake in the morning. It is a lot more pleasant without being woken by an alarm.

Dealing with A Sleepless Night

So, how do you actually deal with those times that you simply cannot fall asleep, no matter what you try.

There are a few ways to do this and we will go through those in due course but first let's go through some facts that you might find interesting.

- Even the act of just lying in bed is helpful when it comes to the body's need to repair itself. So even if you lie awake until three in the morning, you are not completely wasting your time while you are in bed.

- We tend to underestimate how much sleep we have had. Did you feel as though you were awake all night? Sleep studies have shown that we can have sessions of micro-sleep and not even be aware that we were asleep.

  So, while it feels as though you couldn't sleep at all, you probably fell asleep a few times without realizing it.

- The more you stress about not being able to sleep, the less likely you are to be able to sleep.

So basically, that means that you may not be quite as sleep-deprived as you initially thought and that worrying about not being able to sleep is not helpful anyway.

There are going to be times when all the chamomile tea and home remedies in the world are not effective, here is what to try then.

Why Can't You Sleep?

Usually when we can't sleep, there is some sort of reason for it. Are you worried about something in particular or are you just anxious in general? Is there a distraction that is keeping you awake?

Sometimes it can be something as simple as worrying about how you are going to pay a bill. It's a valid concern but not worth losing sleep over. Or maybe you have to remember to buy a birthday card the next day.

How do you switch off worry mode and move to sleep mode? If your worries are keeping you awake at night, something as simple as a little notebook by the side of the bed can be of great help. Write the worries down in this book.

Getting worries down in black and white can be very therapeutic. At the very least, you are letting your brain know that you will be able to deal with them later and not forget about them. If they are written down, you can always deal with them at a later stage.

Is there a physical reason that you cannot sleep? Pain, even a dull, aching pain, can act as a stimulant and keep you awake at night. If you have a back ache or something similar, taking steps to relieve the pain may be enough to help you sleep.

Consider Getting Up

Conventional advice holds that if you cannot fall asleep you should get up and do something else until you feel sleepy again. This can help but only if you do something that is not going to stimulate the mind too much.

Reading a few more chapters in your book by dimmed light, might be helpful, for example. Getting up and playing a computer game, as another example, will not. There are just two rules here – don't do anything that could make you feel even more awake and don't check the time.

Just Lie and Relax in Your Bed

This is another way to handle the problem and it can be more useful than the previous method at times. Enjoy the rest that you are having on the bed. As mentioned before, your body does benefit from the rest, even if you are not sleeping.

If you can just lie there and accept that you might or might not fall asleep, and that either option is okay, this can be a useful trick. If you cannot stop worrying about the fact that you are not sleeping, get up and do something else.

Checking the Time is Counterproductive

We've all done that calculation – if I fall asleep by three o'clock, I can still get five hours sleep and not be a zombie. Clockwatching is only likely to make you more anxious about not being able to sleep.

Why do you feel the need to check the time anyway? So, that you'll know exactly how many hours of sleep you missed? The best outcome is that you'll know how much you missed and feel more tired the next day.

The worst outcome is that the anxiety over the time will keep you awake longer. Neither one is useful for you the next day when you have to get up so just ignore the clock.

Having a Nap

For the most part, I disagree with taking a nap during the day at all times. If you take any more than a half an hour nap, you might wreak havoc with your sleep cycles. And, when you are really tired, a half an hour nap is not going to do that much good anyway.

Where I do agree with napping is if you need to be particularly alert for something. Let's say you need to drive to an appointment or operate heavy machinery. Aside from that, naps should be avoided.

A Note on Sleep Aids

Some people keep over the counter or prescription sleep remedies for those nights when they cannot sleep. I don't think that you should use these on a regular basis but for the odd emergency case they are fine. That said, if you going to take them, take into account that they have a half-life as well.

In other words, the length of time that they are going to be in your system. If you are going to take them at night, sooner is better than later or you could wind up feeling even worse the next day because they won't have left your system before you woke.

Research has shown that sleeping tablets generally allow you to fall asleep only 15 minutes or so before you normally would. For my money, that 15 extra minutes is not worth the REM sleep that you sacrifice as a result of taking these tablets.

Long-term use of sleeping tablets leads to tolerance, meaning that you have to keep upping your dose to achieve the same effects. The side effects include day-time drowsiness, a decline in mental acuity, liver damage, etc.

The main problem with sleeping tablets is that they are notoriously difficult to stop taking if you have been taking them for a while. It will reach a stage where they are no longer effective at making you sleepy but you will be psychologically dependent on them.

In other words, they are not helping you to sleep but if you do not take them, you cannot sleep. If you are not weaned off them properly, rebound insomnia, mood swings and depression can result.

Simply put, the potential risks of taking sleeping tablets outweigh the potential benefits. You are better off suffering a few sleepless nights and reinstating a set sleeping schedule than taking these tablets.

Don't forget to share your thoughts on this book by leaving a review on Amazon.com. It takes just a few seconds.

Discover Scientifically-Proven "Shortcuts" & "Hacks" to Lose Weight FASTER (With Very Little Effort)

For this month only, you can get Linda Westwood's best-selling & most popular book absolutely free – *Weight Loss Secrets You NEED to Know*.

Get Your FREE Copy Here:

TopFitnessAdvice.com/Extras

Discover scientifically-proven tips to help you lose weight faster and easier than ever before. With this book, readers were able to improve their weight loss results and fitness levels. So, it's highly recommended that you get this book, especially while it's free!

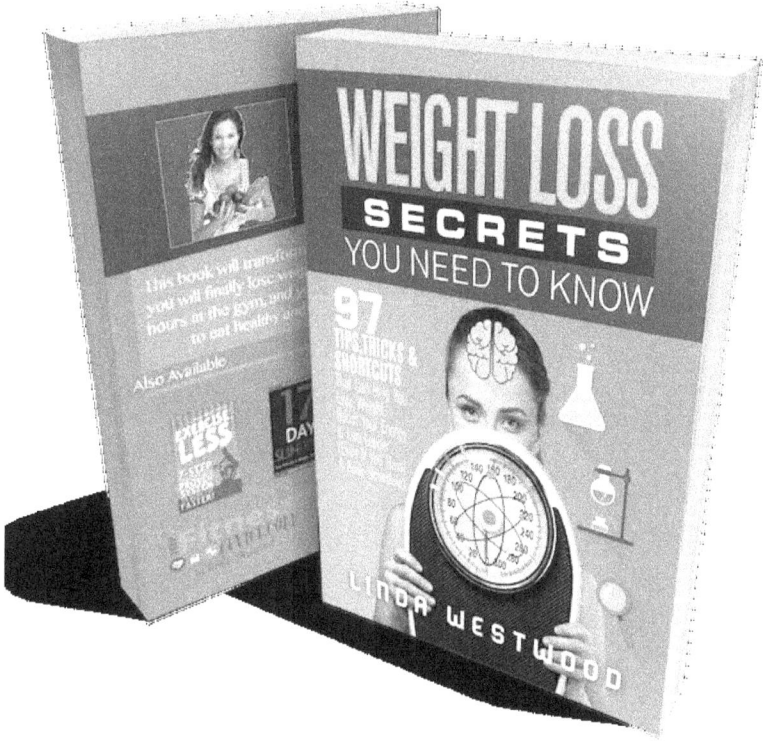

Get Your FREE Copy Here:

TopFitnessAdvice.com/Extras

Conclusion

Well, I hope that you now have a better idea about how you can prevent those sleepless nights.

The key message in this book was to ensure that you get your mind into ideal sleep mode through practicing good sleep hygiene.

By ensuring that you have your bedroom is dark, that distractions are kept to a minimum and that your body is comfortable, you maximize the chances that you will get a good night's sleep.

A lot of things can influence the quality and quantity of sleep that we get – from the coffee we drink to the painkillers that we take.

Identifying why you are unable to sleep is one way in which you can help to minimize the distractions that are keeping you awake.

Once you understand these better, you can create the ideal environment for sleep.

You can reset your sleep cycles and get a full night's rest every night if you are willing to make a few small changes now.

Good luck and see you in your dreams.

Enjoying this book?

Check out our other best sellers!

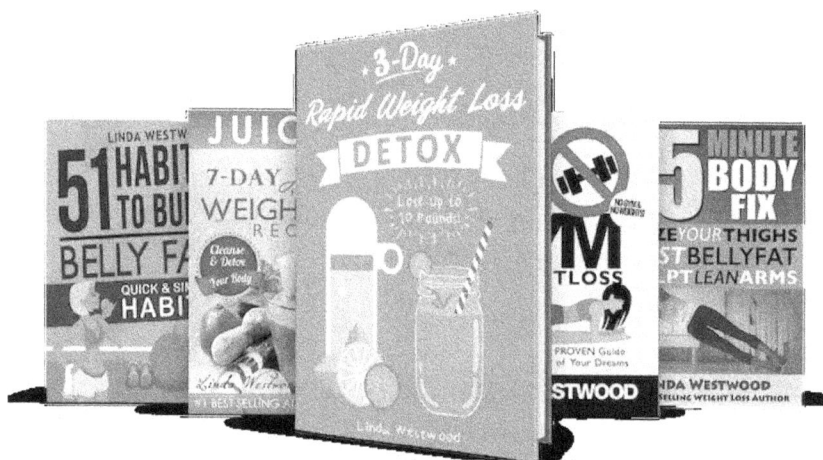

Get your next book on sale here:

TopFitnessAdvice.com/go/books

Final Words

I would like to thank you for purchasing my book and I hope I have been able to help you and educate you on something new.

If you have enjoyed this book and would like to share your positive thoughts, could you please take 30 seconds of your time to go back and give me a review on my Amazon book page.

I greatly appreciate seeing these reviews because it helps me share my hard work.

You can leave me a review on Amazon.com.

Again, thank you and I wish you all the best!